NON-ALCOHOLIC FATTY LIVER DISEASE (NAFLD) COOKBOOK FOR BEGINNERS

Practical Steps, Dietary Interventions, Meal Plans, Medical Insights, And Expert Tips To Combat NAFLD And Restore Liver Health

DR. JACE ZAYDEN

Table of Contents

DISCLAIMER

The information provided in the book is intended for general informational purposes only. The content of this book should not be considered a substitute for professional medical advice, diagnosis, or treatment.

Readers are advised to consult with a qualified healthcare professional for medical advice tailored to their individual circumstances.

The author has made every effort to ensure that the information in this book is accurate and up-to-date at the time of publication. However, medical knowledge is constantly evolving, and new research may emerge that could impact the information presented. The author disclaims any responsibility for any adverse effects or consequences resulting from the use of the information provided in this book.

References or mentions of individuals, products, websites, organizations, or other names within this book are for informational purposes only and do not constitute an endorsement. The author has no affiliations with, and makes no endorsements of, any third-party entities mentioned. Readers are encouraged to conduct their own research and exercise their judgment when considering any external resources or recommendations.

The author and the publisher shall have neither liability nor responsibility to any person or entity with respect to any loss, damage, or injury caused or alleged to be caused directly or indirectly by the information contained in this book. Any reliance on the information within this book is at the reader's own risk.

By reading this book, the reader acknowledges and agrees to the terms of this disclaimer. If the reader does not agree with these terms, they should not use the information provided in this book.

ABOUT THIS BOOK

This "Non-Alcoholic Fatty Liver Disease (NAFLD) Cookbook" is an all-encompassing and essential manual for individuals interested in utilizing dietary interventions to manage and enhance their liver health. This book's organization prioritizes a comprehensive comprehension of NAFLD, with particular emphasis on the pivotal significance of a nutritious diet in both its prevention and management.

The foundational chapters provide a comprehensive explanation of NAFLD complexities and emphasize the criticality of embracing a nutritionally balanced way of life. Significant emphasis is given to the criticality of maintaining a nutritious diet, thereby establishing a solid foundation for the following sections which explore the fundamentals of a diet suitable for NAFLD. The practical implementation of meal planning guidance is ensured, thereby enhancing the accessibility and user-friendliness of the cookbook for individuals who are undergoing dietary adjustments.

This cookbook is exceptional in providing a wide range of gastronomic choices that are specifically designed for individuals who have NAFLD. Every segment, including breakfast, dinner, munchies, and beverages, has been carefully curated with delectable recipes that are also kind to the liver. The dietary recommendations are enhanced in complexity and depth through the incorporation of segments addressing wise culinary techniques, fiber incorporation, lean protein sources, and healthy fats. This empowers readers to make well-informed decisions.

In addition, this cookbook offers a comprehensive perspective on lifestyle modifications by addressing the difficulties associated with dining out, weight management, and physical activity integration. The inclusion of strategies to promote sustained adherence to the recommended dietary adjustments increases the feasibility and viability of the suggested changes to one's lifestyle.

In brief, this "Non-Alcoholic Fatty Liver Disease (NAFLD) Cookbook" is an indispensable reference when it comes to liver health. This manual's thorough structure, educational material, and varied recipe selection render it an indispensable resource for individuals aiming to adopt a proactive approach to enhancing liver health via dietary modifications and lifestyle adjustments.

CHAPTER ONE

Introduction

In recent years, Non-Alcoholic Fatty Liver Disease (NAFLD) incidence has increased substantially, establishing it as a prevalent health concern. NAFLD, which is frequently linked to obesity and metabolic syndrome, is distinguished by the buildup of adipose tissue in the liver of alcohol-free or very infrequent consumers. Although the exact cause of this condition is unknown, it is evident that lifestyle choices, specifically diet, have a significant impact on its development and management. The NAFLD Cookbook is an invaluable resource that provides dietary guidelines and recipes specifically designed to enhance liver health.

NAFLD (Non-Alcoholic Fatty Liver Disease) Comprehension

Before exploring the intricacies of the NAFLD Cookbook, it is crucial to acquire a foundational understanding of the disease. NAFLD comprises a range of hepatic conditions, including non-alcoholic steatohepatitis (NASH), which is characterized by inflammation and potential liver injury, and uncomplicated steatosis, which is characterized by fat accumulation in the liver. In more advanced stages, cirrhosis and liver failure may develop.

The complex mechanisms that initiate NAFLD comprise genetic predispositions, insulin resistance, and lifestyle choices. High cholesterol, obesity, and type 2 diabetes are frequently associated with NAFLD. In contrast to alcoholic liver disease, which is predominantly caused by excessive alcohol consumption, non-alcoholic fatty liver disease (NAFLD) impacts individuals who may not engage in substantial alcohol consumption. This underscores the criticality of incorporating dietary modifications into one's lifestyle.

The Critical Nature Of A Healthful Diet

An essential component in the management of NAFLD entails incorporating a balanced and nutritious diet. In addition to contributing significantly to overall health, a nutritious diet is crucial in preventing the progression of NAFLD. Several dietary constituents have been recognized for their potential to either worsen or mitigate the condition.

Added carbohydrates, highly processed foods, and saturated fats are recognized as contributors to inflammation and the accumulation of liver fat. Conversely, a dietary regimen abundant in lean proteins, fruits, vegetables, and whole grains provides advantageous effects on hepatic health. Berry and verdant green foods, which are abundant in antioxidants, combat oxidative stress, a characteristic frequently observed in NAFLD.

The Cornerstones Of A NAFLD-Complete Diet

The establishment of a liver-friendly diet is facilitated in The NAFLD Cookbook through the promotion of nutrient-dense, whole foods and the restriction of deleterious component consumption. The consumption of omega-3 fatty acids, which are abundant in fatty fish such as salmon and walnuts, is especially advantageous due to their anti-inflammatory characteristics and ability to reinforce liver function. Moreover, electing complex carbohydrates rather than refined ones aids in the regulation of blood sugar levels, thereby mitigating the potential for insulin resistance.

While alcohol does not directly cause NAFLD, it is still advisable to exercise moderation in one's alcohol consumption. However, excessive alcohol consumption can worsen liver injury; therefore, abstaining from or limiting alcohol consumption is recommended to promote liver health.

The cookbook further emphasizes the importance of exercising portion control. Even when consuming nutritious foods in excess, weight gain is a major risk factor for NAFLD. Ensuring that meals are proportionate in terms of protein, fiber, and healthy lipids aids in the regulation of caloric consumption.

Preparing Meals For NAFLD

An essential element of the NAFLD Cookbook is its strong focus on pragmatic meal preparation that is by the dietary requirements of people with NAFLD. The cookbook provides an assortment of delectable recipes that are additionally formulated to support liver health.

Meal planning necessitates the deliberate selection of components and the estimation of portion sizes. The cookbook offers a wide selection of dishes, encompassing breakfast, supper, and refreshments, to guarantee that individuals with NAFLD are presented with a varied and pleasurable menu.

Additionally, it provides recommendations on how to incorporate particular antioxidants and nutrients that are advantageous for liver function.

Meal planning requires that macronutrients, including proteins, carbohydrates, and lipids, be balanced.

The cookbook promotes the consumption of lean proteins, whole cereals, and healthful lipids in moderation, with an emphasis on excluding processed and fried foods. Adopting a balanced approach aids in the regulation of energy intake and promotes metabolic health as a whole.

In summary, the NAFLD Cookbook functions as an all-encompassing manual for individuals seeking to regulate and enhance their hepatic condition via dietary modifications. Comprehending NAFLD, acknowledging the significance of a nutritious diet, laying the groundwork for a liver-friendly eating regimen, and participating in deliberate meal preparation are fundamental measures in advancing liver health.

By applying the principles delineated in the cookbook, individuals can adopt a proactive stance in the management of non-alcoholic fatty liver disease (NAFLD) and promote holistic health.

Breakfast Suggestions For NAFLD: A Nutritious Beginning To The Day

Non-alcoholic fatty Liver Disease (NAFLD) is a common medical condition distinguished by the buildup of adipose tissue in the liver, which is not associated with alcohol intake. The management of NAFLD is significantly influenced by dietary decisions; therefore, preparing a well-planned breakfast is a critical measure in promoting liver health.

A brunch menu for individuals with NAFLD should consist of balanced and nutrient-dense options. It is wise to prioritize whole cereals, fruits, lean proteins, and healthy fats. Oatmeal that has been sprinkled with berries and almonds is a worthy option. Supporting liver function, the soluble fiber in oats assists digestion and helps modulate blood sugar levels.

Complement this dish with Greek yogurt on the side for additional protein and probiotics, both of which promote digestive health.

An additional commendable option is an omelet composed of spinach, tomatoes, and egg yolks. Egg whites offer a superior source of protein devoid of the saturated fat present in the yolk, whereas spinach and tomatoes contribute a beneficial combination of vitamins and antioxidants. Incorporate a portion of whole-grain crostini to enhance

CHAPTER TWO

Dietary Fiber Inclusion

Non-alcoholic fatty liver disease (NAFLD) is a common hepatic ailment distinguished by the buildup of adipose tissue within the hepatocytes; it is not associated with alcohol intake. Dietary interventions are of paramount importance in the management of non-alcoholic fatty liver disease (NAFLD), using fiber incorporation as a pivotal component. A dietary fiber derived from plants facilitates digestion, controls blood sugar, and promotes digestive health as a whole.

In a cookbook devoted to NAFLD, fiber-rich foods must take precedence. Substituting refined grains with whole grains such as quinoa, oats, and brown rice can increase satiety and decrease the risk of blood sugar surges. Incorporate an assortment of vibrant fruits and vegetables into your diet, including citrus fruits, verdant greens, and berries, which are all excellent sources of soluble and insoluble fiber. Soluble fiber aids in the reduction of cholesterol levels, whereas insoluble fiber facilitates digestion by adding substance to the excrement.

Additionally, fiber-rich legumes, including lentils, beans, and chickpeas, are adaptable additives to dishes. In addition to promoting fiber consumption, these plant-based proteins provide an alternative to animal proteins, which may contain excessive amounts of saturated lipids. By incorporating a diverse range of these foods into one's diet, nutrient intake is diversified and liver health is promoted.

Sources Of Lean Protein

Protein is an essential constituent of a well-balanced diet; however, the origin of protein holds considerable importance, particularly for those afflicted with NAFLD. Sources of lean protein are essential for maintaining liver health and symptom management of NAFLD.

Prioritize lean protein options in the cuisine to decrease consumption of saturated fat and enhance overall health.

Fish, specifically fatty fish such as mackerel and salmon, are highly recommended due to their substantial content of omega-3 fatty acids. The anti-inflammatory properties of these essential lipids are advantageous to liver function. Additionally, skinless poultry (including turkey and chicken) is a lean protein source that can be integrated into a multitude of recipes.

Vegetarians and vegans who are looking for protein alternatives should consider plant-based options such as tofu, tempeh, and legumes.

Eggs, and egg whites, in particular, are a multipurpose and protein-rich component that finds application in a wide array of recipes. It is recommended to restrict the intake of red and processed meats due to their frequent content of saturated lipids, which have the potential to exacerbate liver inflammation.

Healthy Fats For Non-Alcoholic Fatty Liver Disease (NAFLD):

While it is advisable to decrease total fat consumption for the management of NAFLD, it is vital to include nutritious lipids in the diet to ensure optimal health. A cookbook for individuals with NAFLD should guide how to make informed decisions regarding the lipids they ingest.

It has been demonstrated that monounsaturated lipids, such as those found in avocados, olive oil, and legumes, promote healthy liver function. Olive oil is a superior option for both cooking and seasoning, whereas avocado can be utilized in salads or as a spread. Nuts and seeds, including almonds, walnuts, and flaxseeds, contribute to fiber consumption in addition to providing healthful lipids.

Chia seeds, flaxseeds, and oily fish all contain polyunsaturated lipids that are an excellent source of omega-3 and omega-6 fatty acids.

The anti-inflammatory properties of these lipids may prove advantageous for those afflicted with

NAFLD. At least twice per week, oily fish can be incorporated into the diet as a palatable and nourishing method to promote liver health.

Restrictions On Processed Foods And Added Sugars

Restricting the consumption of refined foods and added carbohydrates is a fundamental aspect of dietary management for NAFLD. The recipes and guidelines in a cookbook with a concentration on NAFLD should encourage people to make healthier decisions and lessen the strain on their liver.

Frequently concealed in processed foods and sweetened beverages, added carbohydrates can exacerbate NAFLD symptoms by promoting insulin resistance and weight gain. Conversely, for gustatory satisfaction, employ natural sweeteners such as honey or maple syrup sparingly and emphasize the sweetness inherent in fruits.

Restrict consumption of processed foods that are rich in refined carbohydrates, trans fats, and artificial additives. The cookbook may propose alternative options for whole foods, including fresh vegetables, fruits, and whole cereals. Prioritize cooking techniques that maintain the nutritional integrity of ingredients, such as sautéing, barbecuing, roasting, or steaming, over deep frying or excessive oil usage.

Insightful NAFLD Cooking Strategies

A NAFLD cookbook must include advice on intelligent cookery methods to preserve the nutritional value of ingredients and reduce the consumption of unhealthy lipids. The objective is to develop palatable and gratifying dishes that promote hepatic well-being.

Without adding an excessive amount of oil, grilling, roasting, and steaming are all effective cooking techniques for preserving the natural flavors of foods. Instead of high-calorie sauces, grilled vegetables, lean meats, and seafood may be seasoned with herbs and seasonings to enhance flavor.

Olive oil is an example of a heart-healthy oil to use when stir-frying or sautéing. Use sparingly and complement with citrus and seasonings for enhanced flavor. Refrain from deep-frying, as this process may result in the accumulation of detrimental lipids, which can exacerbate inflammation and strain the liver.

Fresh herbs and seasonings can be utilized to enhance the flavor of recipes without requiring an excessive amount of sodium or sugar. This process not only improves the palatability of food but also imparts supplementary health advantages. For instance, the anti-inflammatory properties of turmeric may prove advantageous for those afflicted with NAFLD.

In summary, a cookbook dedicated to Non-Alcoholic Fatty Liver Disease should prioritize the inclusion of dietary fiber, lean sources of protein, and healthy lipids, while reducing the consumption of processed foods and added carbohydrates. Intelligent culinary methods are crucial for guaranteeing that dishes are not only palatable but also beneficial to the liver. By exercising mindfulness and making well-informed decisions while preparing meals, individuals can adopt a proactive approach to managing and enhancing their NAFLD condition.

Complex carbohydrates facilitate the sustained discharge of energy during the morning hours.

When traveling, a smoothie can serve as a nutritious and convenient alternative. Spinach, banana, and a sprinkling of berries are blended with almond milk or low-fat yogurt. In addition to pleasing the senses, this mixture provides the liver with antioxidants and nutrients that are vital to its health.

Keep in mind that moderation is everything and that excessive consumption of added sugars and refined carbohydrates should be avoided.

Choosing whole, unadulterated foods guarantees an initial meal that is abundant in nutrients, thereby providing support for the liver's essential functions.

CHAPTER THREE

Balanced Plate Lunch Ideas To Nourish The Liver For NAFLD

Developing a supper that is conducive to the liver is a calculated measure in the management of non-alcoholic fatty liver disease. The primary objectives of the midday meal should be to supply sustained energy, facilitate satiety, and deliver vital nutrients that support the health of the liver.

One might contemplate preparing a seared salmon salad accompanied by an assortment of vibrant vegetables. Omega-3 fatty acids, which are abundant in salmon, are recognized for their anti-inflammatory attributes.

Incorporating antioxidants and fiber into a dish are bell peppers, verdant greens, and cherry tomatoes. Olive oil, a heart-healthy lipid that supplements liver function, is utilized to dress the salad.

Additionally, quinoa dishes are a fantastic option. Roasted sweet potatoes, black beans, and avocado should be combined with quinoa. Quinoa, being a whole grain, imparts protein and fiber, whereas sweet potatoes furnish a variety of minerals and complex carbohydrates. Black beans provide supplementary fiber and plant-based protein, thereby promoting digestive health as a whole.

Warm-weather eaters may find a stir-fry of vegetables featuring lean chicken or tofu to be a gratifying and nourishing dish. Broccoli, bell peppers, and snap peas are rich in micronutrients and fiber. A protein surge is provided by tofu or chicken without an excess of saturated fat. Reduce the amount of oil used and substitute a ginger-based sauce or soy sauce for flavor.

Adherence to portion control and the selection of foods that promote a well-rounded and varied diet are imperative. Over time, integrating these lunch options that are rich in nutrients into your daily regimen may have a beneficial effect on your liver health.

Dinner Recipes For NAFLD Patients To Support Their Liver

In the late hours of the day, it is essential to conclude it in a manner that is beneficial to the liver. Managing Non-Alcoholic Fatty Liver Disease (NAFLD) requires a conscientious approach that includes dinner as a critical component.

For a dinner that is NAFLD-friendly, lean protein sources, such as fish or poultry, that have been grilled or roasted are outstanding options. Incorporate a substantial portion of roasted or steamed vegetables into their meal to augment fiber consumption and supply vital vitamins and minerals. Sweet potatoes or quinoa are both viable choices for nutritious carbohydrates that contribute to a balanced meal.

Vegetable and lentil curry is a viable option for a plant-based entrée. As a source of plant-based protein and fiber, lentils provide a satiating and nutritious alternative. Incorporate vibrant vegetables such as bell peppers, spinach, and carrots into the curry to increase its antioxidant content. For enhanced flavor, substitute a tomato or coconut milk base for minimal oil.

You may include whole-grain pasta or brown rice in your evening meal selections. Their progressive release of energy from complex carbohydrates aids in blood sugar regulation and promotes healthy liver function. Incorporate a diverse assortment of lean proteins and vegetables into your meal plan to establish a harmonious and nutritious supper.

In the evening, restrict the intake of processed foods, added carbohydrates, and saturated fats. Choose domestic dishes that emphasize the use of fresh, whole ingredients to ensure that your liver receives the most beneficial nutrients.

Indulging Desires While Avoiding Compromise

Snacking may play a pivotal role in the management of non-alcoholic fatty liver disease. Deliberately selected snacks have the potential to sustain energy levels, suppress appetite, and supply vital nutrients that promote the health of the liver.

Nuts and seeds are nutritious options for treats for NAFLD. Chia seeds, walnuts, and almonds are all excellent sources of antioxidants, omega-3 fatty acids, and healthful lipids. These nutrients play a role in the reduction of inflammation and the enhancement of liver function as a whole. Nonetheless, due to the high caloric content of nuts and seeds, portion control is vital.

Berry yogurt topped with Greek yogurt is an additional gratifying and healthful refreshment. Greek yogurt is an excellent source of probiotics and protein, both of which promote digestive health. Berries nourish the liver with antioxidants and impart a natural flavor. Greek yogurt that is pure and unheated will prevent you from consuming added sugars.

Hummus spreads on vegetable skewers constitute a fiber-rich and crunchy appetizer. In addition to being low in calories, carrot, cucumber, and bell pepper spears are also rich in vitamins and minerals. Chickpea-based hummus contributes both protein and healthful lipids to the dish.

Air-popped and mildly seasoned homemade popcorn has the potential to serve as a nutritious substitute for conventional munchies. It is a whole grain that is low in calories and rich in fiber. It is important to exercise caution regarding portion sizes and to refrain from using excessive amounts of butter or oil.

Snacking need not be bland or uninteresting; it can be both enjoyable and healthy for the liver. Incorporate a diverse selection of refreshment options that are rich in nutrients into your daily schedule to promote overall health.

Choices Of Hydrating Beverages For NAFLD Patients' Liver Health

It is even more crucial to maintain adequate hydration when managing Non-Alcoholic Fatty Liver Disease (NAFLD), as this is vital for overall health. Selecting appropriate beverages can make a substantial contribution to enhancing liver function and fostering overall health.

Unsurprisingly, water is the preferred option for hydration. Maintaining adequate hydration permits the liver to carry out its duties, including lipid metabolism, more efficiently. Aim to consume a minimum of eight 8-ounce glasses of water daily. To add a refreshing flavor to plain water, consider infusing it with slices of citrus fruits or cucumber.

Green tea is a beverage recognized for its potential benefits to liver health and antioxidant properties. It contains catechins, which may help reduce fat accumulation in the liver. Nevertheless, exercise moderation; consuming an excessive amount of caffeine is detrimental.

In moderation, freshly strained juices, specifically those derived from fruits such as grapefruit and cranberries, may offer potential health benefits. These fruits contain compounds that may promote the health and function of the liver.

Nonetheless, due consideration must be given to the natural carbohydrates that are contained in fruit fluids.

The administration of herbal infusions, including milk thistle and dandelion tea, is frequently linked to liver support. These teas may potentially possess detoxifying attributes and thus warrant their inclusion in one's beverage selection. Nevertheless, it is recommended that you seek guidance from a healthcare professional before integrating botanical supplements or infusions into your daily regimen.

It is essential to restrict the consumption of sweetened beverages, carbonated sodas, and caffeinated drinks in excessive quantities. These factors may contribute to hepatic fat accumulation and impair liver health as a whole.

In summary, the development of a balanced and hepatoprotective diet necessitates careful deliberation regarding each meal and refreshment.

Every dietary selection, including hydrating beverages, nourishing breakfasts, lunches, dinners, and munchies, can aid in the management of non-alcoholic fatty liver disease. Adhere to a portion control policy and give precedence to whole, nutrient-dense foods to aid your liver in its pursuit of optimal health.

An Anthology Of Liver Health

In recent years, Non-Alcoholic Fatty Liver Disease (NAFLD) has emerged as a significant public health issue, coinciding with the increase in obesity and metabolic disorders. NAFLD, which is distinguished by fat accumulation in the cells of the liver, has the potential to advance into more critical complications, including non-alcoholic steatohepatitis (NASH) and liver cirrhosis. Dietary modifications in particular are crucial in the management of NAFLD among lifestyle modifications.

A NAFLD-specific cookbook provides a pragmatic method for adhering to a diet that is beneficial for the liver.

This book delves into the importance of a cookbook customized for individuals with NAFLD, offering nourishing recipes and advice on weight management, desserts, physical activity, nutritional supplements, and sustainable lifestyle modifications.

CHAPTER FOUR

Recipes Packed With Nutrients To Promote Liver Health: A Culinary Strategy To Confront NAFLD

A crucial aspect of NAFLD management entails incorporating a diet abundant in nutrients that promote the well-being of the liver. A cookbook dedicated specifically to NAFLDs is an invaluable asset in the pursuit of accomplishing this objective.

This cookbook's recipes prioritize components recognized for their beneficial effects on hepatic function, including lean proteins, fruits, vegetables, and whole cereals. These options that are rich in nutrients aid in the reduction of fat accumulation, and inflammation, and the enhancement of liver health as a whole.

Cookbooks dedicated to non-alcoholic fatty liver disease (NAFLD) feature scrumptious and health-conscious recipes, rendering them a readily available option for those grappling with the complexities of liver disease. A diverse array of vibrant fruits and vegetables guarantees an adequate supply of vital vitamins and antioxidants, both of which are indispensable for hepatic oxidative stress resistance. In addition, the integration of lean proteins and healthful lipids contributes to weight management and metabolic marker improvement.

Additionally, the cookbook guides portion control, aiding individuals in achieving a harmonious equilibrium between gratifying meals and sustaining a suitable caloric consumption. By encouraging individuals to manage NAFLD through the foods they ingest in a sustainable and pleasurable manner, these recipes empower them to take responsibility for their dietary decisions.

Preserving Liver Health While Enjoying Delights

Individuals with NAFLD can partake in delectable delights, albeit with moderation, as opposed to conventional wisdom.

The NAFLD cookbook recognizes the occasional consumption of desserts and provides alternatives that are nutritious and gratifying for the liver. These recipes opt to utilize natural sweeteners such as honey or maple syrup instead of refined sugars, while also integrating whole cereals to augment the fiber content.

In desserts intended for individuals with NAFLD, fruits that are recognized for their potential to safeguard the liver are frequently included, including citrus fruits and berries. These alternatives not only fulfill a craving for sweetness but also enhance the nutritional composition of the diet as a whole.

Through meticulous ingredient selection and portion control, individuals can partake in delicacies without compromising the health of their livers.

Eating Out With NAFLD: Making Liver-Friendly Selections From Restaurant Menus

Socializing frequently necessitates dining out, which can be difficult for individuals with NAFLD. The practicality of an NAFLD cookbook is not limited to domestic cookery; it also offers recommendations for selecting nutritious options while dining in restaurants. This particular segment of the cookbook provides valuable guidance regarding menu choices that are by objectives related to liver health.

Important suggestions consist of substituting fried alternatives with grilled or roasted ones, selecting lean sources of protein, and consuming an ample quantity of vegetables. Furthermore, the cookbook provides recommendations regarding portion control and proposes tactics for navigating menus to circumvent concealed origins of added carbohydrates and detrimental fats. Equipped with this information, individuals diagnosed with NAFLD can dine out with assurance, ensuring that social gatherings do not jeopardize their hepatic well-being.

Weight Management And Physical Activity: A Dual Approach To NAFLD Treatment

A comprehensive approach to weight management, which is a cornerstone of NAFLD management, incorporates regular physical activity and dietary modifications. The NAFLD cookbook discusses the significance of weight maintenance and offers recipes that are specifically formulated to aid in both weight reduction and weight sustenance.

It is equally imperative to integrate physical activity into one's daily regimen. With the fitness levels and preexisting health conditions of individuals with NAFLD in consideration, the cookbook guides appropriate exercises. By combining a well-balanced diet with consistent physical activity, this two-pronged strategy promotes weight management and liver health as a whole.

Complementary Methods Of Using Nutritional Supplements To Promote Liver Health

Although the primary focus in managing NAFLD is a well-balanced diet, nutritional supplements may serve as a supplementary tool to aid in the maintenance of liver health. The cookbook guides individuals on the prudent incorporation of supplements, emphasizing those that have been scientifically demonstrated to improve liver function.

Regarding NAFLD, supplements containing omega-3 fatty acids, vitamin E, and milk thistle are frequently suggested. By presenting guidance on suitable dosages and possible drug interactions, the cookbook guarantees the secure and efficacious incorporation of supplements into a comprehensive strategy for liver health.

Long-Term Lifestyle Modification Suggestions: Preserving Liver Health Beyond The Cookbook

Lifelong adherence to liver health is imperative, and the NAFLD cookbook functions as a catalyst for instigating sustained modifications to one's lifestyle. This particular segment of the cookbook provides pragmatic advice and approaches for effortlessly incorporating liver-friendly practices into one's daily routine.

Creating a dietary plan, establishing a regular exercise regimen, and cultivating a supportive environment through community involvement are all recommendations. The cookbook places significant emphasis on the value of consistency and incremental progress, thereby enabling individuals to adopt sustainable lifestyle adjustments that promote the enduring health of their liver.

In summary, a cookbook dedicated to Non-Alcoholic Fatty Liver Disease (NAFLD) functions as an all-encompassing resource for managing the intricacies of liver health, surpassing its mere status as a compilation of recipes. The cookbook offers a comprehensive approach to managing non-alcoholic fatty liver disease (NAFLD), including practical advice on weight management, implementing physical activity, utilizing nutritional supplements, and preparing nutrient-dense meals. Through the promotion of sustained modifications to one's lifestyle, this culinary resource transforms into an indispensable companion during the pursuit of liver wellness. It enables individuals to assume agency over their health and experience a gratifying existence that is conducive to the liver.

Conclusion

In summary, the Non-Alcoholic Fatty Liver Disease (NAFLD) Cookbook serves as a significant asset in the realm of liver condition management and mitigation of its detrimental effects. Achieving an overall improvement in health and liver function necessitates the adoption of a balanced and nutritious diet, given the escalating prevalence of NAFLD on a global scale.

This cookbook functions as an all-encompassing manual, providing a wide range of specialized recipes designed to promote liver health. By placing a strong emphasis on nutrient-dense ingredients and employing mindful culinary techniques, this resource offers individuals coping with NAFLD tasty and practical alternatives. The cookbook's emphasis on whole foods, which are also low in unhealthy lipids and added carbohydrates, is consistent with dietary guidelines that are recognized to promote liver health.

Furthermore, the cookbook includes nutritional information supported by scientific evidence, enabling readers to make well-informed decisions regarding their dietary habits. The dietary plan promotes the inclusion of foods that are beneficial for the liver, including lean proteins, fruits, vegetables, and whole carbohydrates. Conversely, it discourages the intake of refined foods and excessive amounts of sugar. The NAFLD Cookbook adopts a comprehensive approach that encompasses not only the nutritional dimensions of NAFLD management but also the promotion of a sustainable and pleasurable way of life.

The NAFLD Cookbook serves as a pragmatic resource, encouraging individuals to develop a favorable attitude toward food and facilitating the establishment of enduring dietary patterns that promote hepatic well-being. With its emphasis on culinary well-being, it serves as an essential resource for those who wish to manage non-alcoholic fatty liver disease (NAFLD) by consuming nutritious and delectable food.

THE END